THE ART OF COMMUNICATION IN HEALTHCARE

NAVIGATING DIFFICULT CONVERSATIONS WITH PATIENTS AND COLLEAGUES

JASON MILLICAN

The characters and events portrayed in this book are fictitious. Any similarity to real persons, living or dead, is coincidental and not intended by the author.

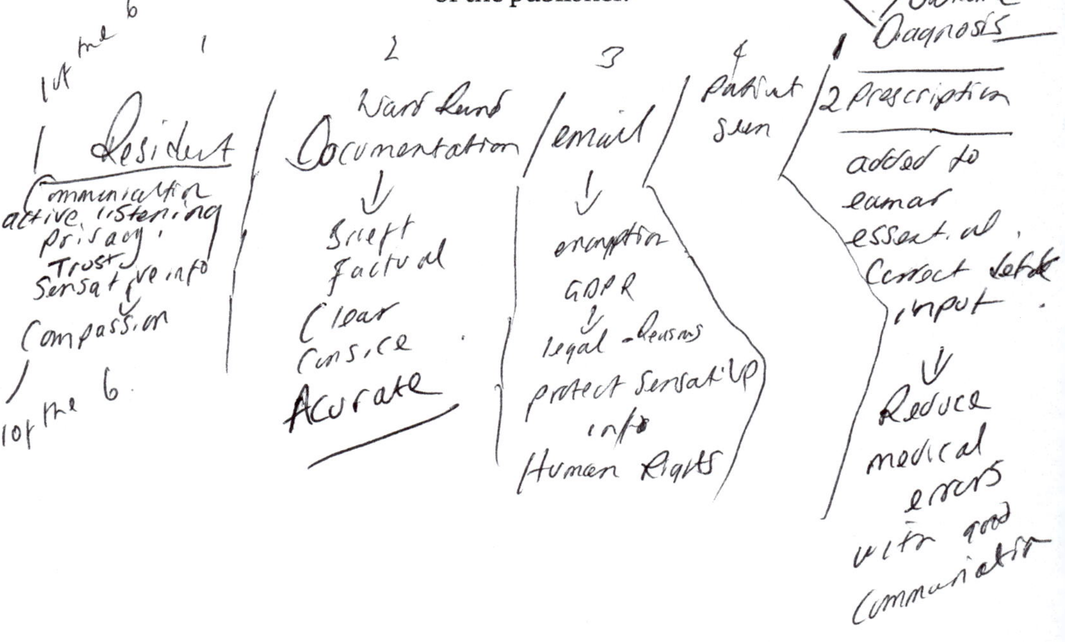

Communication printed copies of Word Fund
— to be stored with team.

CONTENTS

CHAPTER ONE

EFFECTIVE COMMUNICATION FOR HEALTHCARE PROFESSIONALS

Effective communication is a vital component of the healthcare industry. Good communication skills are essential for healthcare professionals to build trust and rapport with patients, provide clear instructions, and make informed decisions. Communication is not just limited to speaking or writing; it also involves non-verbal cues and the ability to actively listen. The quality of communication between healthcare providers and patients has a significant impact on patient outcomes, satisfaction, and the overall functioning of the healthcare system.

The Importance of Effective Communication in Healthcare

Good communication skills are critical in the healthcare industry as they help build trust and rapport between healthcare providers and patients. Patients who feel understood and valued by their healthcare providers are more likely to adhere to their treatment plans, comply with medication schedules, and feel confident in the care they receive. Effective communication also leads to better health outcomes and a lower risk of medical errors.

Benefits of Good Communication for Patients, Healthcare Providers, and the Healthcare System

Good communication not only benefits patients but also healthcare providers and the healthcare system as a whole. Patients who receive clear and concise information are more likely to feel confident in their healthcare decisions and have a better understanding of their conditions and treatments. This can result in improved patient satisfaction and reduced anxiety.

For healthcare providers, good communication skills can improve patient outcomes, increase efficiency, and reduce the risk of medical errors. Health professionals who communicate effectively are better able to understand patients' needs, provide clear instructions, and make informed decisions. Effective communication can also improve the quality of care and lead to better patient outcomes, which can help reduce healthcare costs and increase patient satisfaction.

The healthcare system benefits from good communication in several ways. Improved communication between healthcare providers and patients can result in more efficient and coordinated care, reducing the likelihood of medical errors and improving patient outcomes. Good communication skills can also reduce the need for additional tests, procedures, and appointments, leading to cost savings for the healthcare system. Moreover, improved communication can foster a positive work environment, reduce conflicts, and promote collaboration among healthcare professionals, leading to improved patient care and satisfaction.

Key Elements of Effective Communication in Healthcare

Effective communication in healthcare requires several key elements, including active listening, empathy, clarifying and confirming understanding, providing information, and dealing with challenging situations.

Active listening and empathy are essential in building trust and rapport with patients. Healthcare professionals should be present and attentive when patients are speaking, avoiding distractions, and showing genuine interest in what they have to say. Empathy involves understanding the patient's perspective and feeling, which can help to build a positive and supportive relationship.

Clarifying and confirming understanding involves asking questions and repeating information back to patients to ensure that they have a clear understanding of their condition and treatment plans. Providing information requires clear and concise language, avoiding medical jargon, and using visual aids and handouts to help patients understand complex information.

Dealing with challenging situations, such as difficult patients or emergencies, requires effective communication skills to manage emotions and maintain a professional demeanour. Healthcare professionals should also be prepared to handle sensitive information, maintain patient confidentiality, and respect cultural differences in communication styles.

Communication skills are essential for healthcare professionals to provide quality patient care. Good communication can improve patient outcomes, increase efficiency, and reduce medical errors. Effective communication requires several key elements, including active listening, empathy, clarifying and confirming understanding, providing information, and dealing with challenging situations. Continuous learning and improvement in communication skills are necessary for healthcare professionals to provide the best possible care for their patients.

CHAPTER TWO

VERBAL COMMUNICATION SKILLS

Verbal communication is an essential aspect of healthcare, and healthcare professionals must have strong verbal communication skills to effectively communicate with patients, colleagues, and other healthcare professionals. Good verbal communication skills are crucial in building trust and rapport with patients, providing clear instructions, making informed decisions, and improving patient outcomes.

Active Listening

Active listening is a critical aspect of verbal communication in healthcare. Healthcare professionals must be present and attentive when patients are speaking, avoiding distractions, and showing genuine interest in what they have to say. Active listening involves paying attention to nonverbal cues, such as body language and tone of voice, as well as the words being spoken. By actively listening to patients, healthcare professionals can build trust and rapport, improve patient satisfaction, and provide better care.

Clarity and Conciseness

Healthcare professionals must communicate clearly and

concisely when providing information to patients. They should avoid using medical jargon and technical terms that patients may not understand. Instead, they should use simple, easy-to-understand language and provide visual aids and handouts to help patients understand complex information. Clear and concise communication is crucial in ensuring that patients understand their conditions, treatments, and expectations.

Empathy

Empathy is an important aspect of verbal communication in healthcare. Healthcare professionals must strive to understand the patient's perspective and feelings to build a positive and supportive relationship. Empathy involves acknowledging patients' emotions, responding with empathy, and creating a supportive and non-judgmental environment. By demonstrating empathy, healthcare professionals can build trust and rapport with patients, reduce anxiety, and improve patient satisfaction.

Dealing with Challenging Situations

Healthcare professionals must be prepared to handle challenging situations, such as difficult patients or emergencies. Effective verbal communication skills are essential in managing emotions and maintaining a professional demeanour. Healthcare professionals should remain calm and composed and communicate clearly and respectfully in challenging situations. They should also be prepared to handle sensitive information, maintain patient confidentiality, and respect cultural differences in communication styles.

Verbal communication skills are critical for healthcare professionals to provide quality patient care. Good verbal communication skills can improve patient outcomes, increase efficiency, and reduce medical errors. Effective verbal communication requires active listening, clarity and conciseness, empathy, and the ability to handle challenging situations. Continuous learning and improvement in verbal communication skills are necessary for healthcare professionals to provide the best possible care for their patients.

CHAPTER THREE

NON-VERBAL COMMUNICATION SKILLS

Understanding the Role of Body Language and Non-verbal Cues as a Form of Non-verbal Communication for Healthcare Professionals

Non-verbal communication plays a crucial role in the healthcare industry, and healthcare professionals must understand the importance of body language and non-verbal cues in their interactions with patients. Body language and non-verbal cues can provide information about a patient's feelings, emotions, and attitudes, and can influence the outcome of a healthcare encounter.

Body Language

Body language refers to the non-verbal cues that are communicated through physical movements and gestures. In healthcare, body language can convey a patient's level of comfort, confidence, and engagement in a conversation. For example, crossing one's arms or avoiding eye contact can indicate discomfort or unease, while leaning forward and maintaining eye contact can indicate interest and engagement.

Healthcare professionals must be aware of the body language they are projecting, as well as the body language of their patients. They should strive to maintain open and inviting body language, such as maintaining eye contact, nodding, and smiling, to create a positive and supportive environment. Additionally, healthcare professionals should pay attention to the patient's body language and respond appropriately, such as slowing down or repeating information if the patient appears confused or stressed.

Non-verbal Cues

Non-verbal cues are indirect forms of communication that include gestures, facial expressions, and tone of voice. In healthcare, non-verbal cues can provide information about a patient's level of comfort and understanding. For example, a patient who is tapping their foot or looking at the clock may be anxious or in a hurry, while a patient who is nodding and making positive noises may be indicating agreement and understanding.

Healthcare professionals must pay attention to non-verbal cues to better understand the patient's perspective and needs. They should respond to non-verbal cues by adjusting their communication style and adapting to the patient's needs. For example, if a patient appears anxious or stressed, healthcare professionals may choose to slow down and provide additional reassurance.

Impact of Non-verbal Communication

Non-verbal communication can have a significant impact on the outcome of a healthcare encounter. Good non-verbal communication can build trust and rapport, reduce patient anxiety, and improve patient satisfaction. On the other hand, poor non-verbal communication can lead to miscommunication, increased anxiety, and dissatisfaction with care.

Body language and non-verbal cues play a crucial role in non-verbal communication in healthcare. Healthcare professionals must be aware of their non-verbal cues and the non-verbal cues of their patients to provide effective and compassionate care. By understanding the impact of non-verbal communication, healthcare professionals can improve patient outcomes and enhance the quality of care they provide. Continuous learning and improvement in non-verbal communication skills are essential for healthcare professionals to provide the best possible care for their patients.

Matching Non-Verbal Cues with Verbal Communication for Healthcare Professionals

As a healthcare professional, it is important to understand the impact of non-verbal cues on communication. Non-verbal cues, such as body language, facial expressions, and tone of voice, can greatly influence the outcome of a conversation and should be aligned with the verbal message being conveyed. This is known as matching non-verbal cues with verbal communication.

Body Language

Body language refers to the non-verbal cues that

are communicated through physical movements and gestures. In healthcare, body language can convey a patient's level of comfort, confidence, and engagement in a conversation. For example, crossing one's arms or avoiding eye contact can indicate discomfort or unease, while leaning forward and maintaining eye contact can indicate interest and engagement.

Healthcare professionals must be aware of the body language they are projecting, as well as the body language of their patients. They should strive to maintain open and inviting body language, such as maintaining eye contact, nodding, and smiling, to create a positive and supportive environment. Additionally, healthcare professionals should pay attention to the patient's body language and respond appropriately, such as slowing down or repeating information if the patient appears confused or stressed.

Tone of Voice

The tone of voice refers to the emotional inflexion in a person's speech. In healthcare, tone of voice can convey empathy, professionalism, or even frustration. For example, a monotone or robotic tone of voice can indicate a lack of interest or empathy, while a warm and compassionate tone of voice can indicate understanding and support.

Healthcare professionals must pay attention to their tone of voice, as it can greatly impact the patient's perception of the care they receive. They should strive to maintain a professional and empathetic tone of voice, and respond appropriately to the tone of the patient's speech. For example, if the patient appears stressed or upset, healthcare professionals may choose to use a calming and reassuring tone of voice.

Facial Expressions

Facial expressions refer to the non-verbal cues communicated through the movement of facial muscles. In healthcare, facial expressions can convey emotions such as happiness, sadness, and frustration. For example, a frown or a furrowed brow can indicate dissatisfaction or confusion, while a smile or a relaxed facial expression can indicate happiness or understanding.

Healthcare professionals must be aware of their facial expressions and the facial expressions of their patients. They should strive to maintain a neutral and professional expression while paying attention to the patient's facial expressions and responding appropriately. For example, if the patient appears sad or upset, healthcare professionals may choose to smile and provide additional reassurance.

Impact of Matching Non-Verbal Cues with Verbal Communication

Matching non-verbal cues with verbal communication

can greatly impact the outcome of a healthcare encounter. Good communication, including matching non-verbal cues, can build trust and rapport, reduce patient anxiety, and improve patient satisfaction. On the other hand, poor communication, including mismatched non-verbal cues, can lead to miscommunication, increased anxiety, and dissatisfaction with care.

Matching non-verbal cues with verbal communication is essential for healthcare professionals to provide effective and compassionate care. By being aware of their non-verbal cues and the non-verbal cues of their patients, healthcare professionals can improve the quality of care they provide and enhance patient outcomes. Regular training and continuous improvement in communication skills, including non-verbal cues, are important for healthcare professionals to provide the best possible care for their patients.

Recognizing Cultural Differences in Non-Verbal Communication for Healthcare Professionals

As healthcare professionals, it is important to understand that cultural differences can greatly impact non-verbal communication. Non-verbal cues, such as body language, facial expressions, and gestures, can vary greatly between cultures and have different meanings. This can lead to misunderstandings and miscommunication in the healthcare setting.

Body Language
Body language is a form of non-verbal communication that can vary greatly between cultures. For example, in some cultures, direct eye contact is seen as a sign of respect and attention, while in others, it is seen as aggressive or confrontational. Similarly, gestures such as pointing, nodding, or shaking one's head can have different meanings in different cultures.

Healthcare professionals must be aware of these cultural differences and adjust their body language accordingly. They should strive to maintain open and neutral body language, such as avoiding direct eye contact if it makes the patient uncomfortable, or using culturally appropriate gestures. Additionally, healthcare professionals should pay attention to the patient's body language and respond appropriately, such as slowing down or repeating information if the patient appears confused or uncomfortable.

Facial Expressions
Facial expressions are another form of non-verbal communication that can vary greatly between cultures. For example, in some cultures, smiling is seen as a sign of happiness or friendliness, while in others, it is seen as insincere or fake. Similarly, expressions such as frowning, nodding, or shaking one's head can have different meanings in different cultures.
Healthcare professionals must be aware of these cultural differences and adjust their facial expressions accordingly. They should strive to maintain a neutral and professional expression while paying attention

to the patient's facial expressions and responding appropriately. For example, if the patient appears sad or upset, healthcare professionals may choose to smile and provide additional reassurance.

Gestures

Gestures are another form of non-verbal communication that can vary greatly between cultures. For example, the "ok" gesture, which is a common sign of agreement in many cultures, can have a negative meaning in others. Similarly, the use of hand gestures to emphasize points can have different meanings in different cultures.

Healthcare professionals must be aware of these cultural differences and adjust their gestures accordingly. They should strive to use culturally appropriate gestures, pay attention to the patient's gestures and respond appropriately. For example, if the patient appears uncomfortable with a certain gesture, healthcare professionals may choose to avoid using it.
Impact of Cultural Differences in Non-Verbal

Communication

Cultural differences in non-verbal communication can greatly impact the outcome of a healthcare encounter. Misunderstandings and miscommunication can lead to increased patient anxiety, dissatisfaction with care, and decreased trust in healthcare professionals. On the other hand, recognizing and understanding cultural differences in non-verbal communication can lead to improved communication, increased patient satisfaction, and improved patient outcomes.

Recognizing cultural differences in non-verbal communication is essential for healthcare professionals to provide effective and compassionate care. By being aware of these differences and adjusting their non-verbal cues accordingly, healthcare professionals can improve the quality of care they provide and enhance patient outcomes. Regular training and continuous improvement in cultural competency, including non-verbal communication, are important for healthcare professionals to provide the best possible care for their patients.

Using Appropriate Gestures and Facial Expressions for Healthcare Professionals

Gestures and facial expressions are an important part of non-verbal communication, and healthcare professionals must be mindful of the messages they send through their body language. The right gestures and facial expressions can help to build trust, convey empathy and understanding, and improve the overall patient experience. However, inappropriate gestures and facial expressions can have the opposite effect, leading to misunderstandings and decreased trust in the healthcare professional.

Appropriate Gestures

Healthcare professionals must use gestures that are appropriate for the situation and culturally sensitive. For example, using open and inviting gestures, such as holding the arms open or using the palms of the hands to indicate openness, can convey a sense of trust and comfort. Similarly, using gestures to emphasize a point, such as nodding or pointing, can help to clarify information and encourage active listening.

On the other hand, using gestures that are inappropriate or aggressive, such as pointing or shaking a finger, can convey anger or frustration, and lead to increased patient anxiety. Healthcare professionals must also be mindful of the use of personal space and avoid invading the patient's personal space, as this can make the patient feel uncomfortable and decrease trust in the healthcare professional.

Appropriate Facial Expressions

Facial expressions are another important aspect of non-verbal communication, and healthcare professionals must be mindful of the messages they send through their facial expressions. A neutral and professional expression, such as a slight smile or a neutral expression, can convey empathy and understanding. Additionally, making eye contact with the patient can help to build trust and encourage active listening.

On the other hand, using inappropriate or negative facial expressions, such as frowning, scowling, or rolling the eyes, can convey frustration, anger, or disinterest, and decrease trust in the healthcare professional. Healthcare professionals must also be mindful of cultural differences in facial expressions, as what is seen as a neutral expression in one culture may be seen as a negative expression in another.

Importance of Appropriate Gestures and Facial Expressions

The use of appropriate gestures and facial expressions is essential for healthcare professionals to provide effective and compassionate care. By being mindful of their body language, healthcare professionals can build trust and rapport with patients, convey empathy and understanding, and improve the overall patient experience. Additionally, appropriate gestures and facial expressions can help to clarify information, reduce patient anxiety, and lead to better patient outcomes.

The use of appropriate gestures and facial expressions is an essential part of non-verbal communication for healthcare professionals. By being mindful of their body language and using gestures and facial expressions that are appropriate, culturally sensitive, and empathetic, healthcare professionals can build trust, improve communication, and enhance patient outcomes. Regular training and continuous improvement in cultural competency, including non-verbal communication, are important for healthcare professionals to provide the best possible care for their patients.

CHAPTER FOUR

WRITTEN COMMUNICATION SKILLS

The Importance of Clear, Concise, and Accurate Writing for Healthcare Professionals

Writing is an essential tool for healthcare professionals, as it allows them to communicate important information, share medical reports and recommendations, and document patient information. Writing that is clear, concise, and accurate is essential for healthcare professionals to provide effective care and ensure positive patient outcomes.

Clear Writing

Clear writing is easy to understand, free of confusion and ambiguity, and accurately conveys the intended meaning. In healthcare, clear writing is critical to ensure that patients, family members, and other healthcare professionals understand important information. For example, clear and concise discharge instructions can ensure that patients follow the recommended plan of care and avoid complications after hospitalization. Similarly, clear and concise medical reports can help to ensure that all stakeholders are on the same page and can provide accurate and effective care.

Concise Writing

Concise writing is brief and to the point, focusing on the most important information. In healthcare, concise writing is essential for effective communication, as it reduces confusion and allows healthcare professionals to communicate more efficiently. For example, concise progress notes can help to convey important information promptly and reduce the likelihood of miscommunication between healthcare professionals. Similarly, concise and accurate summaries of medical reports can help to reduce the risk of misinterpretation and ensure that patients and family members receive accurate information about their health status.

Accurate Writing

Accurate writing is factual and free of errors, ensuring that the information being conveyed is correct. In healthcare, accurate writing is essential to ensure that patients receive accurate and effective care. For example, accurate medical reports can help to ensure that patients receive the correct diagnosis and treatment, while accurate medication lists can help to prevent adverse drug events. Additionally, accurate writing can help to reduce the risk of medical malpractice and legal liability.

Importance of Clear, Concise, and Accurate Writing

The importance of clear, concise, and accurate writing in healthcare cannot be overstated. Writing that is clear, concise, and accurate can improve patient outcomes by ensuring that all stakeholders understand important information, reducing the risk of miscommunication and misinterpretation, and ensuring that patients receive accurate and effective care.

Clear, concise, and accurate writing can also help to build trust between healthcare professionals and patients and their families, as it demonstrates professionalism and competence. Additionally, clear and accurate writing can help to avoid medical errors and improve patient safety, as well as reduce the risk of medical malpractice and legal liability.
clear, concise, and accurate writing is an essential tool for healthcare professionals, as it allows them to communicate important information, share medical reports and recommendations, and document patient information. Writing that is clear, concise, and accurate can improve patient outcomes, build trust, and reduce the risk of miscommunication and medical errors.

Healthcare professionals must be mindful of their writing and strive to improve their writing skills to ensure that they provide effective and compassionate care to their patients.

Writing Patient-Centered Medical Records and Progress Notes in Healthcare

Medical records and progress notes are critical components of the healthcare system, as they provide a comprehensive and accurate record of patient care. Toeffective and patient-centred care, it is important for healthcare professionals to write medical records and progress notes that are clear, concise and focused on the patient's perspective.

Patient-Centered Medical Records

Patient-centred medical records are comprehensive records that include all relevant information about a patient's health, including demographics, medical history, and current symptoms and diagnoses. A patient-centred medical record should be written in plain language that is easy for patients and their families to understand and should emphasize the patient's perspective and experiences.

When writing a patient-centred medical-centrededicalalllprofessionals should focus on the patient's health status, current symptoms, and any relevant medical history. They should also document any recommended treatments, medications, and diagnostic tests, as well as any patient concerns or questions. Additionally, healthcare professionals should ensure that medical records are kept up-to-date and accurate, and should document any changes in a patient's health status.

Patient-Centred Progress Notes

Progress notes are brief, daily updates on a patient's health status and progress, and are typically written by healthcare professionals who are directly involved in a patient's care. Progress notes are important for keeping other healthcare professionals informed of a patient's status and for documenting any changes in a patient's condition.

When writing progress notes, healthcare professionals should focus on the patient's health status and any changes in their symptoms or condition. They should also document any treatments or medications that have been administered, and any diagnostic tests or procedures that have been performed. Progress notes should be concise and focused on the most important information, and should be written in a manner that is easy for other healthcare professionals to understand.

The Importance of Writing Patient-Centered Medical Records and Progress Notes

Writing patient-centred medical records and progress notes is important for several reasons. First, it helps to ensure that all relevant information about a patient's health is documented and accessible to healthcare professionals who are involved in their care. This can improve patient outcomes by reducing the risk of miscommunication and ensuring that patients receive accurate and effective care.

Second, patient-centred medical records and progress notes can help to build trust between healthcare professionals and patients and their families, as they demonstrate professionalism and competence. Additionally, writing in a patient-centred manner can help to reduce the risk of medical errors, as it ensures that all relevant information is documented and accessible to healthcare professionals who are involved in a patient's care.

Finally, writing patient-centred medical records and progress notes can help to improve patient satisfaction and engagement, as it allows patients and their families to better understand their health status and the care that

they are receiving.
writing patient-centred medical records and progress notes is critical for providing effective and patient-centred care. By focusing on the patient's perspective and health status, and by writing in a manner that is clear, concise, and easy to understand, healthcare professionals can improve patient outcomes, build trust, and reduce the risk of medical errors. By taking the time to write patient-centred medical records and progress notes, healthcare professionals can ensure that they provide compassionate and effective care to their patients.

Writing Effective Referral Letters and Discharge Summaries in Healthcare

Referral letters and discharge summaries are important components of the healthcare system, as they provide critical information to other healthcare professionals and help to ensure that patients receive appropriate and effective care. Writing effective referral letters and discharge summaries requires clear and concise communication, as well as a focus on the patient's perspective and health status.

Referral Letters

Referral letters are written by healthcare professionals to refer patients to another healthcare professional for further evaluation, treatment, or care. Referral letters should provide a comprehensive and accurate record of a patient's health status, including their medical history,

current symptoms, and any relevant diagnoses.
When writing a referral letter, healthcare professionals should focus on the patient's health status, current symptoms, and any relevant medical history. They should also provide a detailed description of the reason for the referral, including any recommended treatments or diagnostic tests. Additionally, referral letters should be written clearly and concisely, using language that is easy for the recipient to understand.

Discharge Summaries

Discharge summaries are written by healthcare professionals when a patient is discharged from a hospital or other healthcare facility. Discharge summaries provide a comprehensive and accurate record of a patient's health status and care while they were in the facility, and should be written in a manner that is easy for other healthcare professionals to understand.

When writing a discharge summary, healthcare professionals should focus on the patient's health status and any changes in their symptoms or condition while they were in the facility. They should also document any treatments or medications that were administered, and any diagnostic tests or procedures that were performed. Additionally, discharge summaries should provide a summary of the patient's current health status and any recommended treatments or follow-up care.

The Importance of Writing Effective Referral Letters

and Discharge Summaries

Writing effective referral letters and discharge summaries is important for several reasons. First, it helps to ensure that other healthcare professionals have access to accurate and comprehensive information about a patient's health status and care, which can improve patient outcomes by reducing the risk of miscommunication and ensuring that patients receive appropriate and effective care.

Second, writing effective referral letters and discharge summaries can help to build trust between healthcare professionals and patients and their families, as it demonstrates professionalism and competence. Additionally, writing clearly and concisely can help to reduce the risk of medical errors, as it ensures that all relevant information is documented and accessible to healthcare professionals who are involved in a patient's care.

Finally, writing effective referral letters and discharge summaries can help to improve patient satisfaction and engagement, as it allows patients and their families to better understand their health status and the care that they have received.

Writing effective referral letters and discharge summaries is critical for providing effective and patient-centred care. By focusing on the patient's perspective and health status, and by writing clearly and concisely, healthcare professionals can improve patient outcomes, build trust, and reduce the risk of medical errors.

By taking the time to write effective referral letters and discharge summaries, healthcare professionals can ensure that they provide compassionate and effective care to their patients.

Effective communication is a critical component of the healthcare sector. Good communication skills are necessary for healthcare practitioners to create trust and connection with patients, deliver clear instructions, and make educated judgments. Communication is not simply limited to speaking or writing; it also requires non-verbal signs and the capacity to actively listen. The quality of communication between healthcare practitioners and patients has a substantial influence on patient outcomes, satisfaction, and the overall functioning of the healthcare system.

Avoiding Medical Jargon and Using Plain Language in Communication for Healthcare Professionals

Clear and effective communication is essential for ensuring that healthcare professionals provide high-quality and patient-centred care. However, many healthcare professionals use medical jargon and complex language that can be difficult for patients and their families to understand. To provide effective communication, healthcare professionals should avoid medical jargon and use plain language whenever possible.

Medical Jargon

Medical jargon is a type of specialized language used by healthcare professionals that can be difficult for patients and their families to understand. It includes technical terms, abbreviations, and complex phrases that are specific to the medical field. While medical jargon can be useful for communicating with other healthcare professionals, it can be confusing and overwhelming for patients and their families who may not have a background in medicine.

Using Plain Language

Plain language is a type of language that is easy for people to understand and is free of technical terms and jargon. It is used to convey important information clearly and concisely and is especially important for healthcare professionals who need to communicate with patients and their families.

When communicating with patients and their families, healthcare professionals should use plain language to explain medical conditions, treatments, and procedures. They should also avoid using technical terms or abbreviations that may be unfamiliar to the patient. Instead, healthcare professionals should use simple, everyday words that are easy for patients and their families to understand.

Advantages of Using Plain Language

Using plain language in communication has several advantages for healthcare professionals and patients. First, it helps to ensure that patients and their families understand important information about their health status, treatments, and procedures. By using plain language, healthcare professionals can help to reduce confusion and anxiety and improve patient outcomes.

Second, using plain language can help to build trust and increase patient engagement, as patients and their families are more likely to feel informed and empowered when they understand the information being communicated to them. Additionally, using plain language can help to improve patient satisfaction, as patients and their families are more likely to feel that their healthcare provider is compassionate and caring when they use language that is easy for them to understand.

Finally, using plain language can help to reduce the risk of medical errors, as it ensures that all relevant information is documented and accessible to healthcare professionals who are involved in a patient's care.
Avoiding medical jargon and using plain language in communication is critical for providing effective and patient-centred care. By using simple and everyday words, healthcare professionals can ensure that patients and their families understand important information about their health status, treatments, and procedures. By taking the time to use plain language in communication, healthcare professionals can build trust, increase patient engagement, and improve patient outcomes.

CHAPTER FIVE

TEAM COMMUNICATION SKILLS

Collaborating with Interdisciplinary Teams in Healthcare Communication

Healthcare professionals often work in interdisciplinary teams to provide comprehensive and coordinated care for patients. Interdisciplinary teams bring together a variety of healthcare professionals with different areas of expertise, including physicians, nurses, therapists, and other specialists. Effective communication between team members is essential for ensuring that patients receive the highest quality care possible.

The Importance of Collaboration

Collaboration between healthcare professionals is critical for providing patient-centred care. When healthcare professionals work together, they can share information, coordinate care, and provide a more comprehensive treatment plan for patients. Collaboration between team members also allows for the sharing of different perspectives, ideas, and approaches to care, which can lead to improved patient outcomes.

Barriers to Collaboration

Despite the benefits of collaboration, several barriers can make it difficult for healthcare professionals to work together effectively. One of the most common barriers is language, as different members of the team may have different levels of expertise in medical terminology and jargon. Additionally, healthcare professionals may have different communication styles, which can make it difficult for them to effectively share information and collaborate.

Another barrier to collaboration is cultural differences, as different members of the team may have different backgrounds and perspectives that impact the way they communicate. Finally, competing priorities and schedules can also make it difficult for healthcare professionals to collaborate, as they may have limited time to meet and discuss patient care.

Overcoming Barriers to Collaboration

To overcome barriers to collaboration, healthcare professionals need to be proactive in creating an environment that supports effective communication. This can involve creating a shared understanding of medical terminology, using plain language whenever possible, and taking the time to understand the different communication styles of team members.

Healthcare professionals can also take steps to build trust and respect among team members. This can involve creating opportunities for team members to get to know each other, such as team-building activities, and regularly engaging in open and honest communication. By building trust and respect, healthcare professionals can create a culture of collaboration that supports effective communication and patient-centred care.

Collaboration between healthcare professionals is critical for providing high-quality and patient-centred care. By overcoming barriers to collaboration, healthcare professionals can ensure that they are effectively communicating and sharing information, leading to improved patient outcomes. By taking the time to understand the different communication styles of team members, using plain language whenever possible, and building trust and respect, healthcare professionals can create an environment that supports effective communication and collaboration in healthcare.

Building Trust and Creating a Supportive Work Environment in Healthcare

In healthcare, creating a supportive work environment is essential for providing high-quality patient care. A supportive work environment can help healthcare professionals feel valued and engaged, leading to improved job satisfaction, increased productivity, and a more positive patient experience. Building trust among team members is a key aspect of creating a supportive work environment in healthcare.

The Importance of Trust

Trust is essential for effective communication and collaboration in healthcare. When healthcare professionals trust each other, they are more likely to share information and work together to provide the best possible care for patients. Trust can also help to create a more positive and supportive work environment, reducing stress and burnout among healthcare professionals.

Barriers to Building Trust

Despite the importance of trust in healthcare, several barriers can make it difficult to build. One of the most common barriers is a lack of transparency, as healthcare professionals may not feel comfortable sharing information and working together if they are unsure of each other's intentions and motivations.

Another barrier to building trust is a lack of clear communication, as misunderstandings and miscommunications can lead to distrust and conflict among team members. Additionally, cultural differences and different perspectives can also make it difficult to build trust in healthcare, as healthcare professionals may not understand each other's perspectives and approaches to care.

Overcoming Barriers to Building Trust

To overcome barriers to building trust in healthcare, healthcare professionals need to prioritize transparency and open communication. This can involve regularly sharing information about patient care, discussing potential challenges and solutions, and engaging in regular feedback and performance evaluations.

Healthcare professionals can also work to build relationships with each other, creating opportunities for team members to get to know each other and build a shared understanding of each other's strengths and weaknesses. By building relationships, healthcare professionals can create a supportive and trusting work environment that supports effective communication and collaboration.

Creating a Supportive Work Environment

In addition to building trust, creating a supportive work environment in healthcare also involves addressing burnout and stress among healthcare professionals. This can involve providing support and resources for self-care, such as time off and opportunities for professional development, and creating a culture that values and recognizes the contributions of healthcare professionals.

Another aspect of creating a supportive work environment is ensuring that healthcare professionals have the tools and resources they need to provide high-quality care. This can involve investing in technology, providing training and education, and ensuring that healthcare professionals have access to the latest research and best practices in patient care.

Building trust and creating a supportive work environment are critical for ensuring that healthcare professionals can provide the best possible care for patients. By prioritizing transparency and open communication, building relationships, addressing burnout and stress, and providing healthcare professionals with the tools and resources they need to succeed, healthcare organizations can create a supportive and positive work environment that supports effective communication and collaboration in healthcare.

Resolving Conflicts and Promoting Positive Relationships in Healthcare

Healthcare professionals work in a fast-paced and stressful environment, which can lead to conflicts and challenges in communication and collaboration. To provide high-quality patient care, healthcare professionals need to be able to resolve conflicts and promote positive relationships with each other.

The Importance of Conflict Resolution

Conflict resolution is critical in healthcare because conflicts can negatively impact patient care and lead to decreased job satisfaction and burnout among healthcare professionals. Conflicts can arise for a variety of reasons, including differences in opinion, misunderstandings, and cultural differences.

Resolving conflicts in healthcare can help to improve communication and collaboration among team members, leading to a more positive work environment and improved patient care. Additionally, resolving conflicts can help to reduce stress and burnout among healthcare professionals, leading to improved job satisfaction and reduced turnover.

Barriers to Conflict Resolution

Despite the importance of conflict resolution in healthcare, several barriers can make it difficult to resolve conflicts. One of the most common barriers is a lack of communication skills, as healthcare professionals may not have the skills or training to effectively communicate and resolve conflicts.

Another barrier to conflict resolution is a lack of trust among team members, as healthcare professionals may not feel comfortable sharing information or working together if they do not trust each other. Additionally, conflicting priorities and differing perspectives can also make it difficult to resolve conflicts in healthcare.

Overcoming Barriers to Conflict Resolution

To overcome barriers to conflict resolution in healthcare, healthcare professionals need to prioritize effective communication skills and training. This can involve providing training in conflict resolution, active listening, and empathy, as well as opportunities for healthcare professionals to practice these skills in a supportive environment.

Another important aspect of overcoming barriers to conflict resolution is building trust among team members. This can involve regularly sharing information about patient care, engaging in regular feedback and performance evaluations, and creating a culture that values and recognizes the contributions of healthcare professionals.

Promoting Positive Relationships

In addition to resolving conflicts, promoting positive relationships in healthcare is also critical for improving communication and collaboration among team members. Promoting positive relationships can help to create a supportive work environment, reducing stress and burnout among healthcare professionals and improving patient care.

One of the most important aspects of promoting positive relationships in healthcare is creating opportunities for team members to get to know each other and build relationships. This can involve hosting team-building activities and events, encouraging teamwork, and fostering an open and supportive work environment.

Another key aspect of promoting positive relationships in healthcare is valuing and recognizing the contributions of healthcare professionals. This can involve providing opportunities for professional development, investing in technology and resources to support patient care, and creating a culture that values and supports the work of healthcare professionals.

Resolving conflicts and promoting positive relationships are critical for ensuring that healthcare professionals can provide high-quality patient care. By prioritizing effective communication skills and training, building trust among team members, and creating a supportive work environment, healthcare organizations can help healthcare professionals to resolve conflicts, promote positive relationships, and work together effectively to provide the best possible care for patients

Encouraging Open Communication and Feedback in Healthcare

Open communication and feedback are essential for providing high-quality patient care in healthcare. When healthcare professionals have open lines of communication and opportunities to provide feedback, they are better equipped to work together effectively, identify and resolve problems, and improve patient care.

The Importance of Open Communication

Open communication is critical in healthcare because it enables healthcare professionals to share information and collaborate on patient care. When healthcare professionals can communicate openly and effectively, they can more easily identify and resolve problems, work together to provide the best possible care, and respond to patients' needs in a timely and effective manner.

Open communication also helps to promote a supportive work environment and reduce stress and burnout among healthcare professionals. When healthcare professionals feel comfortable sharing information and working together, they are more likely to feel valued and supported, which can improve job satisfaction and reduce turnover.

Barriers to Open Communication

Despite the importance of open communication in healthcare, several barriers can make it difficult to communicate effectively. One of the most common barriers is a lack of trust among team members, as healthcare professionals may not feel comfortable sharing information if they do not trust each other.

Another barrier to open communication is a lack of communication skills, as healthcare professionals may not have the training or experience to communicate effectively in a fast-paced and stressful environment. Additionally, conflicting priorities and differing perspectives can also make it difficult to communicate effectively in healthcare.

Overcoming Barriers to Open Communication

To overcome barriers to open communication in healthcare, it is important to prioritize effective communication skills and training. This can involve providing training in active listening, empathy, and conflict resolution, as well as opportunities for healthcare professionals to practice these skills in a supportive environment.

Another important aspect of overcoming barriers to open communication is building trust among team members. This can involve regularly sharing information about patient care, engaging in regular feedback and performance evaluations, and creating a culture that values and recognizes the contributions of healthcare professionals.

The Importance of Feedback

Feedback is also critical for providing high-quality patient care in healthcare. When healthcare professionals have opportunities to provide feedback, they can share their perspectives and experiences, identify areas for improvement, and work together to make changes that benefit patient care.

Feedback can also help to promote a supportive work environment, as it enables healthcare professionals to share their thoughts and ideas, and feel valued and supported in their work. Additionally, feedback can help to improve job satisfaction and reduce turnover, as healthcare professionals feel empowered to contribute to improving patient care.

Overcoming Barriers to Feedback

Despite the importance of feedback in healthcare, several barriers can make it difficult to provide feedback effectively. One of the most common barriers is a lack of trust among team members, as healthcare professionals may not feel comfortable providing feedback if they do not trust each other.

Another barrier to feedback is a lack of communication skills, as healthcare professionals may not have the training or experience to provide feedback constructively and effectively. Additionally, a culture of fear or a lack of support can also make it difficult to provide feedback in healthcare.

To overcome barriers to feedback in healthcare, it is important to prioritize effective communication skills and training. This can involve providing training in active listening, empathy, and feedback, as well as opportunities for healthcare professionals to practice these skills in a supportive environment.

Another important aspect of overcoming barriers to feedback is building trust among team members. This can involve regularly sharing information about patient care, engaging in regular feedback and performance evaluations, and creating a culture that values and recognizes the contributions of healthcare professionals.

open communication and feedback are essential for providing high-

CHAPTER SIX

THE NEED FOR CONTINUOUS LEARNING AND IMPROVEMENT

Communication is a crucial component of the healthcare industry. It is the foundation of effective patient care and is vital for building trust and creating a supportive work environment. Healthcare professionals must possess strong communication skills to provide the best possible care to their patients.

Verbal communication is an essential aspect of healthcare communication. It involves speaking clearly, actively listening to patients, and avoiding medical jargon. Using plain language and avoiding technical terms can help patients understand their diagnosis, treatment options, and the healthcare process more easily.

Body language and non-verbal cues also play a significant role in healthcare communication. They can convey emotions, and attitudes, and reinforce or contradict verbal messages. Healthcare professionals must be aware of their non-verbal cues and be able to interpret the non-verbal cues of others, particularly in intercultural situations.

Writing skills are also an important aspect of healthcare communication. Clear, concise, and accurate writing is crucial for patient medical records and progress notes, referral letters, and discharge summaries. These documents are critical for the continuity of care and must be easily understood by other healthcare professionals.

Collaboration with interdisciplinary teams is another aspect of healthcare communication. Effective communication between team members can improve patient outcomes, increase productivity, and enhance the overall work environment.
Building trust and creating a supportive work environment are important for healthcare professionals. Open communication and feedback, promoting positive relationships, and resolving conflicts are all critical for creating a supportive and effective healthcare team.
Communication skills are essential for healthcare professionals. They are key to providing quality patient care, building trust, and promoting a supportive work environment. Healthcare professionals must continually strive to improve their communication skills to meet the evolving needs of their patients and their colleagues.

Continuous learning and improvement are essential for healthcare professionals in today's rapidly changing healthcare landscape. As medical knowledge expands and technology advances, healthcare professionals must adapt and develop new skills to provide the best possible care for their patients.
Encouragement for continuous learning and improvement can come from various sources, including personal motivation, peer support, and professional development programs. Healthcare professionals who are passionate about their work and take a proactive

approach to their development are more likely to succeed in their careers and provide better care for their patients.

One way to encourage continuous learning and improvement is through professional development programs. Many organizations offer opportunities for healthcare professionals to attend workshops, conferences, and training sessions that provide hands-on experience and practical knowledge. Attending these programs can provide a wealth of information, as well as a platform to network with other professionals and share best practices.

Peer support is another way to encourage continuous learning and improvement. Working in teams with other healthcare professionals can provide a supportive environment for learning and growth. Colleagues can share their experiences, offer advice and feedback, and help one another navigate the challenges of their careers. By working together, healthcare professionals can encourage each other to stay up-to-date on best practices and improve their skills.

Technology also plays a significant role in encouraging continuous learning and improvement for healthcare professionals. The widespread use of electronic medical records, telemedicine, and other healthcare technology means that healthcare professionals must continually develop their technical skills to stay ahead of the curve.

Finally, self-reflection and self-evaluation are crucial for continuous learning and improvement. Healthcare professionals who take the time to reflect on their practices and identify areas for improvement are better positioned to advance their careers and provide better care for their patients.

In conclusion, encouragement for continuous learning and improvement is essential for healthcare professionals. The healthcare industry is constantly evolving, and healthcare professionals must be prepared to adapt and develop new skills. Whether through professional development programs, peer support, technology, or self-reflection, healthcare professionals must embrace the opportunity to learn and grow in their careers. By doing so, they will be better equipped to provide the best possible care for their patients and stay ahead in their careers.

Effective communication plays a critical role in providing quality patient care. Good communication skills are essential for building trust and rapport with patients, gathering accurate and comprehensive health information, and delivering clear and concise medical information. Communication also plays a key role in promoting positive relationships, resolving conflicts, and collaborating with interdisciplinary teams.

Healthcare professionals must be able to recognize cultural differences in communication and use appropriate gestures, facial expressions, and non-verbal cues to convey empathy and support. Writing skills, including the ability to write patient-centred medical records and progress notes, referral letters, and discharge summaries, are also essential.

Continuous learning and improvement are necessary to maintain and improve communication skills in healthcare. Healthcare professionals must embrace opportunities for professional development, seek peer support, use technology, and reflect on their practices to stay up-to-date and provide the best possible care for their patients.

In summary, communication is a fundamental aspect of providing quality patient care, and healthcare professionals must strive to develop and refine their communication skills to meet the needs of their patients and advance their careers

.

Printed in Great Britain
by Amazon

39086744R00030